GOD HATES ME

Recovering from Religious Trauma, Spiritual Abuse, and an Angry God

IVORY CRUMP

Book production by MysticqueRose Publishing Services LLC

ISBN: 979-8-9915258-0-0

CONTENTS

Letter To Reader .1

Introduction 5

"In the Beginning..." 15

"Obey." 29

"Sinneth Against His Own Body" 41

"Why Hast Thou Forsaken Me?". 47

S.T.E.P.S. 59

Stop 63

Think 71

Evaluate 79

Pivot 87

See 95

Maintaining Your Peace 101

About The Author 109

Letter To Reader

Dear reader,

I wanted to die! I thought I had messed up so bad that my sins were unredeemable. I thought I was cursed by God. I thought God had deserted me, so I had nothing to live for. I was depressed and full of shame. I needed empathy and compassion, but I was met with judgment and harsh criticism. I felt alone and misunderstood.

That is part of my story. I am writing this letter to you as a fellow traveler on a journey that is both deeply personal and profoundly challenging. If you are reading this, it is likely that you have experienced or are currently experiencing the complex and often painful effects of religious trauma. I want you to know that I see you, I hear you, and I understand the depth of your pain.

Religious trauma is a unique form of suffering that is not always recognized or understood by those who have not lived through it. It can stem from a variety of experiences within a religious context, such as spiritual abuse, dogmatic teachings that induce fear or shame, loss of community, or the struggle with doubt and deconstruction of faith. Whatever your experience may be, it is valid, and your feelings are legitimate.

In writing this book, my aim is to provide a safe space for you to explore your experiences, to validate your feelings, and to offer insights and tools that may assist you in your healing journey. I want you to know that you are not alone in this. There are many others who have walked similar paths and have found a way through the darkness.

Healing from religious trauma is a deeply personal process that looks different for everyone. It may involve redefining your spirituality, setting boundaries, or finding new communities that are more aligned with your values and beliefs. Whatever your path looks like, I encourage you to honor your own pace and to be gentle with yourself as you navigate this terrain.

Please remember that it is okay to ask for help, to take breaks when you need them, and to prioritize your mental and emotional well-being. Your journey toward healing is important, and you deserve support and compassion every step of the way.

As you read this book, I hope you find solace in the shared stories, comfort in the knowledge that you are not alone, and strength in the resources provided. May this book be a companion to you as you move forward, helping you break free from religious trauma to find healing, joy, and purpose.

Peace, love, and light.

Ivory Crump

Introduction

I woke up that Sunday morning feeling down and confused. It seemed as if I couldn't get my life together, no matter how hard I tried. It was official: at just 26 years old, I had hit rock bottom.

I felt depressed since I lost my job, house, and car in just three months. 2004 was a rough year. That pain was also fueled by the trauma of the disastrous relationship that I managed to escape. About a year back, in 2003, I started dating a member of the church. He was a young and very handsome minister in training. Being very active in church and a local businessman who owned a barber shop, I was head over heels in love. The infatuation soon came to a screeching halt when, just two months into the relationship, I began to see that he was not at all who he appeared to be.

On a regular basis, he would tell me about messages that he received from God. He was convinced that God was telling him he would be a powerful pastor or that I was cheating on him, or even that others around him were jealous of him. There would even be moments when we would run into a random woman at a grocery store, have a friendly chat, and later, he would claim that the woman wanted him or was turned on by him. I soon realized that this relationship was going off the deep end.

I often found myself afraid to have an opinion. If ever I disagreed with something he said, I was the "rebellious wife" who was going against God for not submitting to him. This was a daily occurrence. Coupled with the cheating accusations and the "God is telling me you're going against Him" statements, it didn't take me long to realize that he was an emotionally abusive narcissist.

I was angry with him for misleading me, but I was even more angry with myself for getting involved with him. I had so much regret about it. After the breakup, I decided to leave the church because I no longer felt comfortable attending the same church as him. Soon, I began going to a church in another city where my cousin was the pastor—I felt safe there, but unfortunately, the drive was always a bit taxing.

That morning, I woke up to the sad reality that was my life, believing I was cursed by God for getting into a relationship that was not His will. I'd begun to feel that way since it ended, but that day, it felt heavier than usual. Reluctantly, I dragged myself out of bed and barely managed to get dressed. I felt like I wasn't capable of driving all the way to my new church, but I also felt like I had to praise God to get back in His good graces. Given how everything went down, I felt like I wasn't in the position to just skip service, so I decided to go to my former church, which was much closer to where I lived. I knew it was a risk, but I was told that my ex no longer attended that church, so I knew I wouldn't run into him there. It was better than not going at all.

I got into the beaten-up old car I bought from my cousin dirt-cheap and headed to the church. As I drove, I turned on the radio to the gospel station, and "Make Me Over" by Tonex began to play. I typically liked this song, but that day, it was hitting me like a ton of bricks. After listening for a few minutes, I turned it off and finished my drive in silence.

When I arrived, I walked up to the front door of the church, feeling burdened. I felt like I was weighed down when I entered, and was surprised to be greeted by some of the members, many of whom I had not seen since I left. I was immediately thrust into a deep feeling of worship as the praise team's melodic voices and tambourines filled the church. Almost subconsciously, I threw my hands up and started running around the church, clapping my hands and thanking God. The feeling was beautifully overwhelming.

As I rounded up my second lap around the pews, the pastor called me up to the front of the church. The sudden sound of my name being called over the loudspeakers stopped me in my tracks. I turned to face the front of the church, and there was the pastor with a mic in his hands, staring me down. He had recently condemned me for leaving the church in the first place and had taken it upon himself to send messages to my sister, trying to get her to convince me that I was out of God's will. I felt conflicted being back, but thought I'd be welcomed and perhaps even embraced.

As I stared at him from a distance, the look on his face suggested I had no choice but to walk up to the altar. Reluctantly, I walked to the front of the church, dreading what he was going to say. Without even looking, I could feel the eyes of all the church members follow me as I approached him. Standing at the foot of the platform, I looked up at the menacing pastor.

"Raise your hands," he demanded.

Confused by the command, I stood still.

"Raise your hands to receive the Word of God," he repeated.

I felt like I had to comply with his instructions, so I did as I was told. A wry smile appeared on his face. He looked to the congregation while placing his hand on my shoulder.

"This child has lost her way!" he informed them, "But we are all capable of redemption!"

"Amen!" the church shouted in response.

He looked back to me, and with the mic close to his lips, said, "Either you're going to attend our church and be a part of this family. Or you go there to that church and stay there. Find your place and get in God's will! Amen?"

"Amen!" the church responded. In that moment, I felt a cool wind sweep over me. I felt as though I were naked in front of everyone. I felt exposed, embarrassed, and ashamed. Was I perfect? No. But was attending another church a sin?

The pastor looked back at me and shook his head in disappointment. He removed his hand from my shoulder and turned back as he began preaching to the church.

Slowly, I turned from the altar and shamefully found my seat, wondering what I had done wrong. I was confused, and I felt worse than I did when I walked through the doors. Was choosing to leave this church and attending another so bad?

This is just one of the many painful experiences from my past that contributed to my religious trauma, but as I look back on it, I realize how much wisdom I've gained because of those moments. For instance, being on the receiving end of such harsh criticism under the guise of religion taught me to show others grace and think carefully about what I say and how I say it.

Each of those painful experiences has helped shape me into the spiritual life coach that I am today. One of the philosophies that I teach is, "life is a school, and experience is your teacher," meaning everything that you go through in life is meant to teach you a lesson. There's no such thing as coincidence, so the things that happen in your life are meant to happen. We learn and grow from our life experiences.

A big part of my healing was finding the silver lining in all the painful experiences from my past. I turned my pain into purpose. Healing from child abuse, depression, and religious trauma motivated me to help others who are also experiencing issues around spirituality, such as religious trauma and spiritual awakening. This is where I discovered my ultimate purpose.

Being able to help others was paramount to me, but in order to do that, I had to be trained and educated. Without hesitation, I began looking for opportunities that would allow me to work and learn at the same time. Luckily, an opportunity came my way in 2013, and I started working in the mental health field as a peer support specialist. Since then, I have worked in substance abuse, employment support, and applied behavior analysis therapy.

As I worked and trained, I was also receiving life-changing spiritual mentorship from Reginald Martin. It was through his guidance that I not only completed my healing but gained the confidence I needed to take the leap and help others. I moved powerfully through life coach training and received my certification in 2021.

The skills I developed through my work experience in the mental health field and my personal experiences were easily integrated into my new profession as a spiritual life coach. Fast forward to today, and I've been able to help dozens of people navigate their path of self-discovery while fulfilling their purpose and overcoming limiting beliefs associated with religious trauma. This is all done through my proven framework, S.T.E.P.S.

S.T.E.P.S. is rooted in my philosophy of "transform your beliefs, transform your life." The way religious trauma thrives in your life is through the way you've unintentionally wired your mind. Strict religious upbringing, spiritual abuse, and exposure to harmful religious teachings have wired your brain in a way that perpetuates trauma and negative patterns in your life. When you grow up in a strict religious environment or are exposed to spiritual abuse, your beliefs about yourself, the world, and the Divine can become distorted. These distorted beliefs can lead to feelings of guilt, shame, fear, and unworthiness. For example, you might believe that you are inherently sinful or that you must adhere to rigid rules to be worthy of love or salvation. These beliefs can create a constant state of anxiety and self-doubt, impacting your mental and emotional well-being. To transform your life, it is essential to first transform your beliefs. This involves examining the beliefs that have been instilled in you and determining whether they serve your highest good. It requires challenging deeply ingrained beliefs and replacing them with more empowering and compassionate ones. The S.T.E.P.S. method helps you to rewire your mind and realign your thoughts to deal with and heal from your trauma powerfully. As you transform your belief system through the S.T.E.P.S., you will be led to an outward transformation in your life.

S.T.E.P.S. stands for **Stop**, **Think**, **Evaluate**, **Pivot**, and **See**. With these five steps, you will be able to work through the mental or emotional challenge that has you stuck. This is the exact framework I used to regain control of my life, restore my self-esteem, and build a more powerful union with the Universe. Now, I am giving this framework to you as a tool to use on your journey to healing.

CHAPTER 1

"In the Beginning..."

It was early summer and I was in the backyard playing with my older sister and cousin as the sun smiled warmly upon us. Our house sat on an acre of land so our backyard was spacious enough for us to roam freely. There was a red barn on the far right corner of the yard where my dad kept his lawn mower and other outdoor equipment and tools. There was an old well on the left that was out of use, so my parents covered it to keep us safe. We enjoyed running around in the backyard. That day, we were playing the game "What Time is it, Mr. Fox?" The game requires one person to stand a significant distance away from the other players with their back turned. The other players ask, "What time is it, Mr. Fox?" The person calls out a number and the other players take that many steps toward them. The first player to reach the "fox" tags them, then the "fox" begins to chase the other players. Whoever the "fox" tags first becomes the "fox" for the next round. My cousin was the "fox," so she stood at the far end of the yard while we stood by the house.

"What time is it, Mr. Fox?" I yelled to my cousin. "Three o'clock," she replied, and I stretched my tiny legs as far as I could reach in three giant steps. "What time is it, Mr. Fox?" I yelled again. "Seven o'clock," she shouted back, so I hopped seven steps. Just as I was taking my last step, my mother called out in a booming voice, "Ivory, you're being too loud!" I was so startled that I almost lost my balance. I turned around and saw my mom standing by the backdoor. "Okay, mom, sorry," I said and turned around to resume the game as she walked away. "What time is it, Mr. Fox?" I exclaimed, and my cousin shouted, "Five o'clock!" I took five steps in her direction, and then asked for the time again. No sooner had I gotten the words out of my mouth than I heard my mother calling out from the backdoor. "Ivory, come here!" she said. I froze for a few moments before turning to face her. I could tell by her glare that she was angry. I began walking slowly, cautiously, and begrudgingly in her direction, trying to prolong the steps to reach her. I was afraid. "Is she going to hit me?" I wondered. Her eyes were steadied on me as I approached her. As I made my way up the steps to the door, she growled, "Get in this house. I told you, you were being too loud," and yanked me by my arm. My heart was pounding as she led me into her room and slammed the door behind us. She let go of my hand and walked toward her dresser. She grabbed two of my dad's neckties and a t-shirt from the dresser drawer. She said she was going to teach me a lesson. I stood by the bed, frozen, anticipating what was to come. She tore off part of the shirt and used it to gag my mouth and then used one necktie to tie my feet together and the other to bind my arms. She went back to the dresser and pulled out a long black belt. She walked toward me and pushed me onto the bed and began to beat me with the belt. I cried as I felt the lashes from the belt stinging my skin. I wanted to say "I'm sorry," but I couldn't speak. I laid there helpless, wanting it to be over. When she finally stopped, I remained there sobbing. "Next time I tell you to be quiet, you better listen, stupid," she yelled.

It wasn't my first time being beaten, and certainly not the last. I knew it hurt, but I was too young to understand that it was abusive behavior. I accepted it as normal: you do something bad, you get beaten—plain and simple. That was how she raised me and I didn't dare question her because it would lead to getting hit more. I was taught that questioning an adult's actions, especially hers, was disrespectful. She said that God commanded children to obey their parents and that the Bible said, "spare the rod, spoil the child."

I was born in a small rural town in North Carolina where I lived with my mother, father, and older sister. My parents were conservative Christians and we attended a Baptist church where my father served as a minister. Later, when he transitioned from being a minister to pastoring a church, he joined the Presbyterian denomination. I followed him and became a member of his church, but my mother remained a Baptist.

My parents divorced when I was in the 6th grade and this had a significant impact on me because it was a major life change and I didn't know how to cope with it. My mother insisted that we live with her and my father complied so we had no choice but to move with her from the rural community to an apartment in the city. I began to notice how controlling my mother was after we moved and this made me depressed. I saw a drastic difference between my mother and my father's parenting style. My mother didn't allow us to spend time with friends. We couldn't even go to the playground in the apartment complex often because there were boys in the neighborhood and we might commit the sinful act of having sex, according to her. We were relieved when my dad came to get us on weekends because he was more lenient and gave us choices rather than dominate us. He took us to watch movies, skate, bowl, enjoy waterparks—whatever we wanted to do. We could talk openly and honestly with him, and he gave constructive feedback and shared his wisdom. My dad became a safe space where I could vent about the situation with my mother. He expressed how harsh and unfair her behavior was, and that it bothered him that she wouldn't allow us the choice to live with him.

Meanwhile, things grew from bad to worse between me and my mom, and I wanted so badly to escape from her. One day, my sister and I were getting ready for bed when my mother came into our bedroom and started fussing at her for a reason I can't remember. As my mom was leaving our room, she said to me, "You better get in bed before you get in trouble too," and walked out. I looked at my sister, shrugged my shoulders in puzzlement, and said, "I didn't even do anything." My mom rushed back into our room asking me to repeat what I said. "Mom, all I said was that I didn't do anything," I pleaded as she lunged at me, smacking me repeatedly. She went wild, swinging at me and I tried my best to shield myself from the blows. This went on for what seemed like an eternity until she stopped suddenly. I looked up as she stood there panting heavily with a crazed look in her eyes. She stood there for a few more minutes just looking at me before leaving the room. I felt hurt, sad, and enraged—I hated her with a passion.

These moments of her lashing out became more frequent, and after a beating, she would claim we somehow disrespected her. She would justify her beatings by saying, "The Bible says to honor thy mother and father." I found myself afraid to respond when she spoke to us for fear of punishment.

Relief came in my 10th grade year when my mother agreed to let us live with my father after years of begging. Finally, freedom! I could go to football games and spend time with my friends. We took frequent trips to Atlanta and visited Virginia and other places. I could go to parties and hang out with my cousins.

The trauma from my mother's mistreatment and justification through religion caused me to begin to explore other religions and spiritual philosophies. Thanks to my newfound freedom, I allowed myself to question Christianity and eventually renounce it altogether. My family made it clear that they did not support my decision and would often try to convince me to come back. I understood that many of them just wanted the best for me, but if how my mother behaved was true Christian behavior, I wanted no part of it.

There are far too many horrific stories like my own where individuals are hurt in the name of religion or spirituality, leading to lasting psychological and emotional scars. One testimonial involves Jim, a 35-year-old male who was raised by a single mother. Jim's mother became close with the pastor at the church they attended when he was a child. When Jim entered his pre-teen years, the pastor asked Jim's mother if he could mentor him. The pastor began to pick Jim up each week to spend time with him. What Jim's mother didn't know was that the pastor would molest Jim when he took him away. Jim struggled with depression and shame since then but never told anyone what happened. Another testimonial involves Shameka, a 21-year-old African American female. She was raised in the Christian religion and the church she attended as a child followed a legalistic doctrine. As a result, her parents were strict, controlling, and would not allow her to spend time with friends or engage in extracurricular activities because they considered them to be "worldly." Instead, Shameka was forced to attend church excessively because her parents thought that was being a good Christian. In addition, Shameka was physically abused by her parents. Shameka moved into her own place at the age of 18 to escape her parents' abuse, legalism, and controlling behavior. She stopped going to church and distanced herself from the Christian religion when she moved out. Shameka has struggled with ruminating thoughts about death and going to hell since then.

Spiritual abuse occurs when a person uses religion or spirituality to control, manipulate, or cause psychological, sexual, or physical harm to us. The abuse can be caused by a religious/spiritual leader, member of the religious/spiritual community, parent, family member, or significant other. Often, the perpetrators gain a benefit from abusing others—whether it be power, money and material items, or even pleasure. They prefer a system of hierarchy where they are on top of the chain with little to no accountability so that their abusive actions will go unchecked and they can use their authority to thwart and demonize you if you question them. These perpetrators will twist religious doctrine and spiritual philosophy to justify their behaviors and control you. While reverence for religious and spiritual leaders is common, it can lead to abuse when we follow them blindly or believe they are beyond reproach—leaving the door wide open for hypocrisy, deceit, coercion, immorality, and exploitation.

Spiritual abuse triggers the body's stress response system and it becomes overactive due to prolonged exposure to the dysfunctional environment, which can lead to chronic stress and other mental health issues, such as anxiety and PTSD. Studies have also shown that it affects the areas of the brain responsible for learning, memory, perception, and decision-making. In addition, it hinders our emotional stability and causes irregularity in our fight-or-flight response system.

Overcoming spiritual abuse begins with leaving the abusive environment and distancing yourself from the perpetrator so they are no longer in control. Severing your ties to the toxic relationship gives you freedom to reestablish your sense of autonomy and self-identity. It creates a safe space for you to heal and reflect without fear of being manipulated or coerced. The separation also makes room for you to form new, healthy relationships and explore different spiritual practices that help you grow and establish independence. This is how I was able to escape from my mother's oppressive grip and find liberation, peace, and safety.

****

After graduating from high school, I moved to Atlanta to attend Bauder College, where I got my associate degree. A few years later, I went back to school at Langston University where I obtained my bachelor's degree. I had become interested in black empowerment as a teenager and started reading books like The Miseducation of the Negro, The Autobiography of Malcolm X, and Message to the Black Man. By the time I got to Langston, I would only wear traditional African attire and I had even legally taken an African name. My French professor was a Nigerian woman, and she encouraged me to participate in the study abroad trip to West Africa she was coordinating, and I accepted.

I prepared myself to travel to Ghana and Togo in 2002 with my professor and a group of students. The day to leave for the motherland finally arrived and my roommate dropped me off at the airport. I hopped out of the car and hurried inside with my luggage in tow and spotted the trip coordinator waving at me as she stood with the other students. I joined the group smiling and waited until the boarding call was finally made and we hurried to line up. I found myself sitting next to a student I didn't know because the trip coordinator assigned our seats. I gave a friendly smile and greeted her as I approached, placed my carry-on in the compartment above, and slid into my seat. I conversed with my neighbor and some of the students sitting nearby. We talked about our majors, where we were from, and why we decided to take this trip. After conversing for a while, I turned my attention to the movie showing on the large tv in the airplane. Eighteen hours later, after two plane changes and a two-hour layover, we arrived in Accra. We hustled our way through the airport and stepped out into the open air. I felt like I was dreaming. "We're finally here," I thought as I took in the scenery.

Traveling to my ancestral home was a life-changing experience. We went to a market where we saw vendors selling everything from beautiful African fabric and jewelry to traditional attires. We also visited Kumasi, a rural city in Ghana—the greenery and kind residents made it a memorable visit. The most impactful part of the trip was visiting what the natives referred to as "castles," where the slave trades happened. Standing face-to-face with "the door of no return"—the very threshold where they loaded Africans onto ships and transported them to America during the slave trade—was overwhelming to say the least.

The coordinator was a devout Christian so she took us to an African church as part of our cultural immersion experience. When we got to the church, she was asked to introduce the minister who would be preaching. She went up to the podium, took the mic in her hand, and in a loud thunderous voice, said, "When God calls you, you must go." I started trembling inside and my heart began to beat violently out of fear as I thought, "Oh no, is God calling me?" Up until I went to Africa, I knew I wanted to empower the black community, but I didn't know in what way I would make the contribution. At that moment, I began to believe that my calling was to be a minister and missionary due to my religious upbringing. I was convinced that the coordinator was talking about me and I didn't want to disobey God. In addition to my religious upbringing, the economic disparity I saw weighed heavily on my heart as I realized that what we considered low income in America equated to a lot more than poverty in Ghana. So, I started to believe that being a missionary was the way to give back to the community. I rededicated my life to Jesus after returning from Africa, then I graduated and moved back home. I returned to NC with high hopes for the future and a new zeal for God, not knowing that tragedy awaited me.

CHAPTER 2

"Obey."

I was enthusiastic about my faith in Jesus so I joined the church my sister was attending and went as often as possible after returning to NC. I was introduced to baptism of the Holy Spirit, speaking in tongues, prophesying, laying of hands, deliverance, and spiritual warfare. Coming from a traditional Baptist and Presbyterian background, this was all new to me. This was the first time I heard people talk about hearing the voice of God. I found it all fascinating and intriguing.

The pastor would often warn us that we must be careful about making decisions so "we would stay in

God's will." He would often say that that's the safest place to be. He also warned about the consequences of getting out of God's will. He preached that you wouldn't be blessed by God if you went against the plan He had for you. He stressed that we should pray and ask God what His will was before making any decisions.

I wanted so desperately to know what God's plan was for me. I would often pray and ask God for direction because I didn't want to be punished for going against Him. The problem was I wasn't sure how to recognize God's voice. I was taught the flesh was weak and the heart was deceitfully wicked, so how was I supposed to know and trust when God was speaking to me? I didn't want to be deceived by my flesh.

I shared with my pastor that I believed I was called to be a minister and missionary. He advised me to pray and ask God if it was His will. He explained that there had been things he wanted to do in the past but realized that God had a different plan for him.

We were having a special service that week at the church and my pastor encouraged me to attend because the guest speaker was a prophetess. He suggested that perhaps God would speak through this prophetess and confirm it was His will for me to be a missionary. So, I attended the service as directed. After preaching, the prophetess began to call people up to the front of the church to give them a prophecy from God. Suddenly, she looked at me and called me up to the front of the church. She said to me, "I see the way that you are dressed (I had on traditional African attire), and God said you are going to Africa. I see a vision of you ministering to children there." I was both excited and amazed that God had spoken through this woman who didn't know me from a can of paint.

I was on a high after receiving that prophecy because I finally knew what God's plan was for me. Things were going great. I landed my first job after graduating from college and bought my first house. I believed all these things were blessings from God because I was in His will. Amidst all these great things, I also started dating a guy from my church and was head over heels in love.

The way our romance started was like a beautifully orchestrated twist of fate designed by the hands of God. I was part of the church media team and the pastor invited me to see a play at a production studio a few hours away. He instructed me to meet him at the church and when I pulled into the parking lot, there he stood with my soon-to-be boyfriend, Billy. The pastor walked over to my car and leaned in the window to ask if Billy could ride with me and I agreed. Billy got into the car and immediately suggested we pray before leaving. He asked if I could say a prayer especially for him because his ex-wife had an affair and he was trying to heal from all the terrible things she and her mother had done to him. We locked hands and bowed our heads and prayed that God would protect us as we traveled to the studio. I also asked God to mend his heart and help him heal from the trauma he had experienced. Then, we headed to the studio.

Billy didn't say much on the way, instead, he read his bible while I listened to worship music on the radio. We arrived two hours later and went inside to take our seats. Midway through the play, I was enjoying myself when Billy leaned over and said he was going outside. I turned to him and said,

"Okay," and he looked at me like he expected me to follow him. I turned my focus back to the play and he headed outside, but eventually came back. When we returned to the car after the play was over, he told me he had walked out in the middle of the play because he misjudged it as worldly, but came back after he realized he was wrong. I shared how I found the play entertaining and would like to come back when they were having another production, and we made light conversation as we returned to the church. When we arrived at the church, he thanked me for the ride and invited me to go into the church to pray. Billy and I prayed for about an hour, then bid each other goodnight and went home.

Two days later, he called me and explained that he got my phone number from my brother-in-law. He told me he called me because he believed God told him I was to be his wife. He seemed to be as passionate about God as I was: we were both in the choir and praise team and he was also a minister in training, so I believed him and we began officially dating.

Our relationship was going great, we continually shared our love for God, regularly prayed together, and often spoke about our dreams of preaching the gospel. As time passed, he shared more and more details about his previous marriage. He held back tears as he explained that his ex cheated twice: once with a member of the community and then with his landlord. He said that he divorced her immediately after he found out. My heart ached for him as I listened to his story. I truly felt bad for him and even told myself I'd do what it takes for him to trust me.

One day, we went out for an afternoon drive. The sun was shining as worship music played on the radio. It was a rather serene day as I drove down the quiet road. Billy seemed peaceful and content as he sat in the passenger seat. We soon struck up a casual conversation about me being part of a rap group back in the day. I made mention of the group's talent manager at the time, a nice woman in her 40s. I immediately noticed Billy's demeanor change as I mentioned her name. His shoulders drew back and he stared at me with a quiet rage.

"What?" I asked, shifting my eyes from the road to him and back to the road again.

Billy's eyes smoldered as he began connecting imaginary dots. He claimed that the man his ex-wife cheated on him with knew my former manager. According to Billy, that meant that I must have also slept with this guy. I couldn't believe it! Was he accusing me of cheating on him with a man that I didn't even know? I attempted to reassure him that it wasn't true and perhaps he was having trust issues due to his former wife's infidelity. That only seemed to enrage him more as he began to berate me and claim I was lying. He insisted God had told him, so there was no use in me lying to him about it.

Unfortunately, situations like this would soon become the norm. He would often share with me that God told him that certain people were against him and praying for his downfall. Sometimes, when we went out, Billy would also claim that women we encountered were making advances toward him. He often talked about how God would send him messages and he had a grandiose idea that he was going to be a mega preacher.

I loved Billy, but I was starting to question some of his behavior. His superiority complex began to spiral out of control. Not to mention, he would flip-flop about whether he actually heard God say we were supposed to get married.

During service one Sunday, the pastor announced that our congregation had been invited to a special service by the prophetess and her husband who had preached at our church previously. On the day of the service, her husband delivered the sermon and then began to give prophecies to people afterward. I was sitting with Billy and we watched as he called people up one by one to the front of the church, and told them what he felt God was telling him. All of sudden, he looked at me and Billy, and motioned for us to come up. We looked at each other in surprise and walked to the front of the church and stood in front of him, wondering what he was about to tell us. The prophet looked at us and said, "Hold hands." Billy and I linked hands, and he said, "God wants y'all to get married. You two are supposed to serve in ministry together." Billy and I turned to each other and began to laugh partly in shock and partly in excitement. My doubts about our relationship began to fade as we made our way back to our seats because of the prophecy. "It *must* be God's will for us to be together," I thought.

Billy's accusations toward me became more frequent after that, and he would have outbursts whenever there was a difference of opinion and he lectured me about being a rebellious wife and how it was my place to submit to him. His paranoia about people conspiring against him continued to grow. The accusations and paranoia became too much for me and I began to realize that it was not God's will for me to be in this toxic relationship. I wanted to end it, but I had to find the right timing so it wouldn't set him off. So, I talked with my dad about the situation and he advised me to discuss what was going on with my pastor and ask him to meet with me and Billy. I talked with my pastor and he understood and agreed to meet with us. The following Sunday, I told Billy I wanted to talk with him and the pastor so we headed into his office. The pastor greeted us when we walked in, and I told Billy that I wanted us to reach an understanding. I asked him if he had heard God speak to him directly and tell him that we were supposed to get married, and he said no. I told him God had not spoken to me directly as well, so we agreed to end the relationship. I was relieved.

With a clean break from Billy, it seemed as if all was right with the world, but suddenly, things started to go downhill. I lost my job within months of us breaking up and this was the beginning of my financial troubles. Next, my car got repossessed, and then, I had to foreclose on my house. I was convinced all these things were happening because I'd been out of God's will by getting into that toxic relationship. I believed that I had forfeited the prophecy I had received as a punishment from God. I felt that my life was ruined by that one bad decision. I expected bad things to happen to me, so each time I experienced an unfavorable circumstance, it reinforced my belief that I was being punished by God. I felt confused and I was afraid of making any major decisions out of fear of making the wrong one. Because of this, I was stagnant and unable to progress.

Religious fear can manifest as indecision and paralysis, as was the case for me. It can cause anxiety, panic attacks, ruminating thoughts, and night terrors. Some are tormented with a fear of going to hell and facing eternal damnation. Others fear that they have committed a sin that God will not forgive. Fear of the great tribulation can cause you to be afraid to leave the house. Religious fear can cause you to isolate yourself from the outside world out of fear of being influenced by evil. It will cause you to keep secrets from your family and religious community out of fear of being judged. While some live with a fear of being attacked by Satan and/or demons.

I've shared my experience with fear from religious trauma, but religious fear looks different for everyone. A former client shared that she would wake up in the middle of the night in a panic, afraid she was rejected by God because she had been told by various members from the religious community that she was not a child of God. Another individual confided in me that she struggled with severe anxiety due to ruminating thoughts about burning in the lake of fire for eternity. From another testimonial, a person recalled being petrified ever since learning about hell, rapture, and the end times as a child. In another testimonial, an individual expressed their fear of going to hell because of their addiction.

Fear is a basic human response triggered by a perceived threat. With religious trauma, the threat can be divine punishment, eternal damnation, or judgment and rejection from the religious community. Fear activates the part of the brain that processes emotions, releasing stress hormones, such as cortisol and adrenaline. This activates the fight-or-flight response. Prolonged fear from religious trauma can cause changes to brain structure and functioning that result in issues such as anxiety and PTSD.

Religious fear impacts your entire life because it influences your beliefs, which in turn influences your behavior and decision-making. Living in a constant state of fear prevents you from fully embracing life because you are guarded and always in protection mode. You have little to no trust in anyone or anything. You prefer what is comfortable and predictable and avoid taking risks and uncertainty. You become a prisoner to your fears until you are ready to face them head-on.

At the time, I certainly was not in a place to face these fears head-on and I continued to suffer silently in my prison. As every area of my life seemed to fall apart right before my eyes, I never imagined this trauma would also impact my sex life.

CHAPTER 3

"Sinneth Against His Own Body"

After the relationship with Billy, I convinced myself that it was safer to date someone with whom I was already familiar, so I tried rekindling a connection with an ex-boyfriend. I quickly realized that my wounds were too fresh and I needed time to get over the heartache. The thing that bothered me the most about the situation was that I had compromised my relationship with God by engaging in sex with Billy. I knew it was a sin, but I told myself that it was okay because we were planning to get married. I closed my heart off from everyone because I didn't want to get hurt again and decided I was no longer going to date, but rather focus on growing closer to Jesus.

I didn't want to lose my connection with God after leaving the church Billy and I had attended, so I started to attend my cousin's church. Even though I was isolating myself, I couldn't help but notice one handsome guy who would show up to service every Sunday. Dave was his name, and he was just my type—tall, slender, and he seemed to be a devout Christian. I had such a huge crush on him, but I only admired him from a distance. I was intent on maintaining my relationship with God and not giving in to temptation. One day, as I was leaving the church, I passed by Dave on my way out the door. As I walked toward my car, I heard someone calling my name. I recognized the voice and my heart began to beat rapidly, "Oh my God, it's him! It's Dave," I thought to myself. "Just keep walking," I told myself, and hurried off to my car as if I hadn't heard him. I often wonder what he thought as I briskly walked to my car, ignoring his call. I was so afraid of disappointing God that I refused to even speak to a man I found attractive.

The trauma I had experienced from the toxic relationship and the fear my mother instilled in me caused me to run away from Dave and anyone else who tried to get close to me. I remember hearing preachers give warnings about dating people who were not Christian, but I felt that Christian men could be just as bad as the ones who weren't saved, as proven to me by Billy. On top of that, I was still haunted by the belief that I was being punished by God and I felt so low about myself that I didn't think I had anything to offer anyone.

Rigid religious rules and guidelines can make it difficult to date and form intimate relationships. Many religious leaders use scriptures about fornication and sexual immorality to teach congregants that sex outside of marriage is sinful. Some even condemn masturbation, causing a sense of guilt. In addition, many religious leaders teach that heterosexuality is the only acceptable form of relationship, and homosexuality is considered an "abomination." People with same-sex attractions are expected to deny their feelings and force themselves to be with the opposite sex or live a life of celibacy.

Setting a standard that expressing sexuality is only acceptable within marriage leads to sexual repression where we are disconnected from and ashamed of our sensuality and sexual desires. It can also cause those who engage in sex to feel extremely guilty and like they need to hide it from others. When we are taught these things as children, it can make the changes that we go through as we develop even more difficult because of the shame. Never truly feeling comfortable with our sexuality can cause severe challenges, such as anxiety, erectile dysfunction, and vaginismus when we do try to have sexual relationships. It is crucial to recognize and address the profound impact these teachings can have on our psychological and sexual well-being.

I remember a time when a young woman confided in me as she recalled how her first sexual encounter as a teen turned into a nightmare when her mother walked in on her and her boyfriend. She recounted how her mother became enraged and physically beat her, locked her in her room for 48 hours, and then forced her to "repent" aloud to God for her sins. Unfortunately, stories of physical punishment and mistreatment surrounding sex and religion are commonplace. I recall watching a YouTube video where a young man shared that his family and church community tried to discourage him from being homosexual. They advised him to pray and fast and ask God to take away his sexual desires. The young man says that he followed their advice, but his desires did not go away. When he finally decided to embrace his same-sex attractions, he was excommunicated from the religious community.

Thanks to my conditioning, from age 27 to 33, I didn't date, but there was one platonic friend, Henry, with whom I enjoyed spending time. We would go to restaurants, movies, and the park, or just hang out at his place and watch TV. I found his company very comforting, although he had no idea about the painful relationship from my past or how much his companionship meant to me during that time. One day, we were sitting on the couch at his place watching television. We were nestled closely together, and I rested my head on Henry's shoulder. I looked up at him and our eyes locked, and without a second thought, our lips met in a kiss. It felt right, and one thing led to another, and soon we found ourselves making love. It was undoubtedly satisfying but when it was over, reality set in. What should have been a sweet and pure intimate moment between close friends was overshadowed by my guilt. "Oh no! I broke my vow to God!" I thought and burst into tears right next to Henry. He knew how much my faith meant to me because we'd had a conversation about me being celibate in the past. He placed his hand on my shoulder and tried to console me, but it was too late—the damage was already done. Not too long after, we had a chance to talk about it and he shared with me that what happened between us was not bad and it was destined to happen. I was feeling better about the situation by then, however, I still felt that I had committed a sin against God.

I felt like there was no justification for my actions and I would be punished. It was all becoming too much to bear. Although I was functioning, I was in a bad place mentally. Still, I was trying to heal my heart and pick up the pieces of my life, but just when I thought things couldn't get any worse...I finally reached my breaking point.

CHAPTER 4

"Why Hast Thou Forsaken Me?"

I was still trying to overcome the thoughts that I was being punished by God and was a failure, so I thought a change of scenery would be good. I had developed an interest in church planting so I began reading a number of books on the subject. One of the authors I was reading on the subject taught at Fuller Theological Seminary in Pasadena, California. I looked up the school and found out they offered a certificate in church planting, and I got excited. "Wow, I can get a master's degree in divinity with a concentration in church planting!

This is awesome!" I thought. I applied to the program, and was accepted, to my delight—and that settled it…I was moving to California.

The first thing on my agenda to prepare for the move was to figure out where I was going to live. The school had several apartment communities to choose from and they had a database with all the available units. There was even one for those who were looking for roommates in their units. So, I searched the database and found a female who lived in a three-bedroom and was looking for two roommates. I called to inquire about the apartment and a young woman named Jane answered the phone. Her tone was friendly and warm, and I got a good impression from the conversation, so I told her I was interested in rooming with her. She seemed excited and said she would start the process.

A few weeks later, I got a call from a woman named Kim, who said she had gotten my name and information from Jane. Jane had informed her that I'd be their third roommate. Kim sounded very worked up about something so I listened as she continued to talk. She said that as Jane was showing her around the apartment, they went to the refrigerator, and when she opened it, the refrigerator was full. Seeing that there was no more room in the fridge, Kim asked Jane, "What about me and Ivory? Where are we supposed to put our stuff?" "Why would she mention me and put me in the middle of their conflict? I don't have anything to do with it," I thought to myself, but I continued to listen as she went on to say that Jane got upset by her question. She went to the housing office later and overheard Jane telling the resident assistant that she no longer wanted to room with us. At this point, I'm thinking to myself, "Oh no, there's already drama and I haven't even gotten there yet." I listened as Kim bashed Jane's character, claiming that she had no right to judge us for wanting "space in the fridge," and it must be a sign that Jane would have been a horrible roommate. She then suggested that she and I move into a two-bedroom together so we could still be roommates. Thinking that Jane had completely changed her mind about having roommates, I agreed.

Later in the week, I received a call from Jane who was very apologetic. She said she was sorry that things didn't work out, as she heard Kim and I were going to move into a different apartment. She explained that she didn't want to live with Kim after meeting her because she had a very rude attitude, but she was glad I had found a place to stay. Again, I listened as I had with Kim and remained silent until she finished. I figured there was no point in mentioning that Kim had told me she was the one who didn't want to room with us. I simply thanked her and wished her well before hanging up.

Kim called me again later in the week to find out when I would be coming to California. I told her the date, and she began to tell me that she already had furniture for the living room and dishes in the kitchen, so all I needed was a bed and furniture for my room. She asked what I was going to do about getting a bed and I told her I would handle furnishing my room after I got there. She went on to say she found a bed for sale on Craigslist and could go ahead and get it for me if I was interested. I figured it would take a lot off of my plate so I said, "Fine." She then asked how I was going to get to campus, and I told her I would catch a cab, but she immediately insisted on picking me up, so again, I said, "Fine."

Kim came to the airport to pick me up on the day I arrived as promised. We made small talk on the ride back and decided to stop and get something to eat. She took me to a Thai restaurant that, according to her, served really good food. As we ate dinner, we talked about our spiritual beliefs and I mentioned that I believe drinking is a sin and she politely disagreed. I didn't think anything of it and our conversation continued normally. Toward the end of our meal, Kim revealed that she had borrowed her friend's car to pick me up, thus we needed to go to their house to return it. Kim's friend and her roommate were having dinner when we arrived, so we sat at the table with them and chatted for a while before leaving. I felt truly welcomed in California and thought this would be a great experience. Kim and I seemed to get along pretty well and she even introduced me to more of her friends on campus the next day, albeit briefly. When I returned home later that day, Kim was sitting in the living room cwhen I walked in and said she needed to talk to me. "What's up?" I asked. "Honestly," she said in a deep tone, a tone I was not used to, "I want to talk about your behavior." I gave her a puzzled look and she let out a sigh as if she were gravely disappointed. "You've been acting real judgemental toward me and my friends," she said with an accusing look on her face. "What?" I responded in disbelief.

She went on to say that when we went to her friend's house to return the car, I turned my back to them because they were drinking. She also claimed that when she saw me on campus and introduced me to her friends earlier, I was rude for leaving so soon without much conversation. She even accused me of thinking that I was better than everyone because of how I was looking at them. With each accusation, she grew louder and more aggressive. "No!" I said defensively. "I didn't mean to offend you or your friends. I didn't realize anyone was offended!" I tried to reason with her. Nonetheless, she kept insisting I was being judgmental. It was clear that the conversation wasn't going anywhere and I was getting frustrated about the accusations, so I just suggested that she not introduce me to any more of her friends.

It hadn't occurred to me at the time, but Kim was showing similar traits to both my mother and Billy, and the red flags grew one by one. There were three more incidents where she confronted me in anger about something I supposedly did wrong. I finally decided this was not an environment I could thrive in. I decided that the best thing for me to do was move out.

In order to move out without being fined for breaking the lease, the resident assistant advised me to try to resolve the issues with my roommate. The man reminded me that we were a Christian community and seminary students which meant I needed to learn how to resolve conflict. It just so happened that when I got home that day, Kim confronted me yet again with a new issue. She wanted to know why I hadn't been talking to her lately and accused that I was causing tension in the house. As she started lashing out at me, I began to tremble with anxiety. It was hard for me to breathe as I stood there listening to her rant loudly. I began to feel weak as I stood there bearing the full weight of her verbal onslaught, so I leaned on the counter for support. The energy in the room felt weird and nasty as she continued to rage. I was relieved when she finally finished so I could leave the room. I rushed out of the door and down the steps and just as I stepped outside, I began to feel a sharp pain in my stomach. The pain was so severe that I dropped to my knees. I forced myself to breathe slowly and once I recovered, I immediately went to report the incident to the resident assistant. Fortunately, I was released from the lease agreement and allowed to move into my own apartment.

I was glad to be in a space of my own so I could have peace, but the peace was short-lived as things spun out of control. I was angry and hurt about what happened with Kim which caused me to be conflicted because, after all, *doesn't God want us to forgive?* I needed time to heal so I tried my best to avoid Kim whenever I saw her on campus. Try as I might, she would always find me and approach me as if she was trying to force me to speak to her. I would do my best to ignore her as she went on her tirade about how I messed things up for her.

I moved to California for a fresh start, but it seemed that a dark cloud in the form of Kim had followed me from North Carolina. I was so stressed that it got to the point where I couldn't sleep. I would wake up in the morning and begin my day worrying about bumping into Kim, and sure enough, I would run into her several times. Each time, she'd dive into her barrage of complaints and accusations. I'd flee to my class, try to clear her from my memory, go home, attempt to study, attempt to sleep (and fail), and start it all over again. Day after day, I'd move through this horrible cycle praying that she would just disappear, but she never did.

What disturbed me the most was how she reminded me of my mother. The accusations, the guilt-tripping, the shouting, it was like I was back in my childhood home, closing my eyes and praying it would all end. Only now, I was an adult. I shouldn't be feeling this way. I shouldn't be made to feel so small, and I most certainly should not be letting this affect me the way it was. But unfortunately, it was. I felt small. I felt tired. I felt hopeless. Day in and day out, the stress and emotional weight of it all pulled me further and further into a depth of despair I thought I'd climbed out of. I was afraid to bring it up to anyone else for fear of ridicule. I was an adult, after all, I should be able to handle this on my own. Yet, I could not. Eventually, I hit my breaking point. The stress and sleep deprivation led to me having a nervous breakdown. I became delusional—one of my classmates saw me wandering around campus and called 911.

A nervous breakdown is a term used to describe a state where a person becomes so overwhelmed by stress that they become incapable of functioning in day-to-day life. Things had mounted and I had reached my breaking point and had to be hospitalized. While in the hospital, I learned that I was suffering from trauma and depression. I had deep unresolved issues that went all the way back to my childhood and the relationships with Billy and Kim had exacerbated the problem.

In the book, *The Body Keeps the Score*, Kolk writes, "…trauma is not just an event that took place sometime in the past; it is also the imprint left by that experience on mind, brain and body. This imprint has ongoing consequences for how the human organism manages to survive in the present."[1] Psychological wounds, like physical wounds, can grow worse if not treated, and this was the case for me. I didn't know what depression or trauma was before I entered the hospital. I knew that I felt bad about myself, but I didn't have a language for what

---

1. Bessel Van der Kolk, *The Body Keeps the Score: Brain, Mind, and Bodyin the Healing of Trauma*. (New York: Penguin Books, 2015), p. 21

I was experiencing, nor did I know I needed help. Kolk goes on to say that he learned through his experience working in a psychiatric hospital that, "…more than half the people who seek psychiatric care have been assaulted, abandoned, neglected, or even raped as children, or have witnessed violence in their families."[2] Unresolved trauma can cause severe psychological and physical problems that affect your daily functioning, relationships, and overall quality of life.

I had my first experience with therapy while at the hospital where I met one-on-one with a counselor and attended group sessions, and I continued to work with a counselor once I returned to North Carolina after being discharged from the hospital. At first, it was awkward for me to open up and share my mental and emotional struggles with others because I had never done so before. African Americans are taught to be strong and tough in order to survive and endure the harsh realities of racism and socioeconomic disadvantages so being emotionally vulnerable is considered weakness and mental illness is taboo. As a result, many suppress

---

2. See Footnote 1

their mental and emotional pain as a means of survival. As I continued therapy, I began to release the anger that I had been holding inside for so long. I was able to heal from the depression, anxiety, low self-esteem, shame, guilt, and suicidal ideations and deconstruct the toxic religious beliefs.

Being hospitalized was the beginning of my healing journey because it led to me getting the therapy I so desperately needed. Now, it's your time to heal. The next section will walk you through how to heal from your religious trauma. For additional support, you can reach me at ivorycrump.com.

CHAPTER 5

S.T.E.P.S.

S.T.E.P.S. (Stop, Think, Evaluate, Pivot, See) is the framework I designed to help you reframe your negative thoughts and beliefs to overcome your trauma. Reframing is when you take a negative thought and change it to something positive. S.T.E.P.S. is a breakdown of that reframing process that will help you challenge the negative beliefs you have about yourself that are caused by religious doctrine or things said and done by religious leaders, family, or community members. As you start to reframe those negative thoughts, you will begin to feel better about yourself and the world around you. Your beliefs and thought patterns influence your emotions and decisions which result in how you feel about yourself, the world, and the outcomes in your life. So, when you change those beliefs, your perception of reality will change. My motto is: Transform your beliefs, transform your life.

The neurons in your brain send out signals called neurotransmitters to tell your body what to do every time you have a thought or complete an action. These neurons are connected through pathways that run from one area of the brain to another. When we replay the same thoughts, emotions, and actions constantly, a protective coating is formed over a pathway to strengthen the connection between neurons. As these pathways become stronger and stronger, we get "stuck" because certain behaviors and thought patterns become automatic. The good news is we are capable of creating new pathways by learning new ways of thinking and acting which weakens the old pathways. This is what makes S.T.E.P.S. so powerful.

I used reframing to overcome the negative beliefs about myself which influenced how I perceived the world. I thought I was cursed and had ruined my life beyond repair, and there was no hope for me. I was drowning in a sea of despair, shame, guilt, and regret. Once I reframed my thoughts, I was no longer depressed. Now, I am sharing this framework with you because I want you to overcome religious trauma too.

Please keep in mind that, depending on the severity of your trauma, for example, sexual abuse, you may need to seek therapy in addition to using this framework. This is a tool to help you deconstruct the toxic religious programming that you are struggling with.

Okay, let's take a deep dive into the next few chapters where I break down the S.T.E.P.S. formula!

CHAPTER 6

Stop

According to a research study conducted by Julie Tseng and Jordan Poppenk,[3] the average person has more than 6,000 thoughts per day, so the chatter in your mind is constant. In simple terms, our thoughts are the messages we tell ourselves about the things we experience from moment to moment. As we process sensory information, our brain fires signals that create thoughts, keeping our minds continually active. Our thoughts are how we perceive reality and what we decide to do about it.

---

3. Jordan Poppenk & Julie Tseng, "Brain meta-state transitions demarcate thoughts across task contexts exposing the mental noise of trait neuroticism," *Nature Communications* 11, 3480 (2020): p. 7, https://doi.org/10.1038/s41467-020-17255-9

There are two levels to our thoughts—the conscious and subconscious level. An iceberg is a common analogy used to explain these levels. Most of the iceberg is underwater so we don't see it—this represents the subconscious mind. We only see the tip of the iceberg, which represents the conscious mind. Conscious thoughts are those we are aware of that come when we focus on an object or task in the present. Reading a book or solving a math problem are examples of the conscious mind at work.

Subconscious thoughts are the automatic, impulsive processes that come from memories and past experiences that are stored beneath our level of awareness. They influence our decisions and behaviors without us realizing it. The subconscious mind includes habits, instincts, and routines that have become second nature to us through repetition, such as brushing your teeth and tying your shoes. It also stores emotions, biases, and beliefs formed from our past experiences.

Beliefs are things we accept as true, either based on our personal experiences or what people tell us. Past experiences, beginning in childhood, shape our belief systems. As we interact with others and our environment, we draw conclusions about what we experience, and those conclusions form our belief systems. Beliefs influence our thoughts, emotions, decisions, and behaviors—including negative self-talk. Since beliefs are stored in the subconscious mind, we often do not even realize that they are impacting what we think and do.

With religious trauma, our beliefs and thoughts are influenced by our past religious experiences. I was haunted by the horrifying belief that I was being punished by God because of the legalistic doctrine I was taught at my former church. Anytime I experienced an adverse circumstance, I thought it was an act of divine punishment. Trauma changes the brain and the way we see the world by telling us our survival is being threatened, so now, we must rewire our minds and brains to tell our bodies that we are safe because the threat is gone. Overcoming religious trauma requires us to deconstruct and dismantle the harmful beliefs that come from toxic religious/spiritual doctrine and/or things that have been said or done to us by religious/spiritual leaders, family, or community members. Deconstructing and reframing our thoughts begins with stopping and quieting our minds to bring our thoughts under control.

The first step in the S.T.E.P.S. is Stop. You must stop by pausing in order to get a clear vision of your negative self-talk. You must be conscious of what you need to change in order to reframe your thoughts. They will continue to pour negativity over anything you do moving forward unless you stop them. Negative self-talk can cause us to feel out of control, but *Stop* is the process of regaining control by centering ourselves. Centering brings us to a state of calmness and stability so that we can think clearly. We can use breathing exercises and visualization to do this.

Yoga teaches that if we can control our breathing, we can control the mind. Doing breathing exercises, also called breathwork, redirects our focus from the negative self-talk to our breath. Breathwork can be used to increase our energy, regulate our mood, slow our heart rate, lower our blood pressure, and calm us down. Using a slow, deep breathing exercise to calm and center ourselves helps stabilize the autonomic nervous system by deactivating the sympathetic nervous system or fight-or-flight response, which allows the parasympathetic nervous system to tell our brains and bodies that we can relax because we are safe. Our breathing is controlled by a part of the parasympathetic nervous system called the vagus nerve. The vagus nerve also controls digestion, cardiovascular activity, and heart rate. We engage the vagus nerve when we practice slow, deep breathing, which in turn slows our heart rate, decreases our blood pressure, and has a calming effect on our bodies.

In order to fully *Stop*, we must also visualize. Visualization is when we close our eyes and use our imagination to picture an image that makes us feel safe, calm, and relaxed. Someone may imagine they are sitting on the beach watching the soothing waves of the ocean, while someone else may picture themselves walking through a meadow—everyone's safe place will look different. When we practice visualization, our brains respond to the image in the same way it would if it were happening in real life. So, if we imagine something that calms us and makes us feel safe, then our brains will send a signal throughout our bodies that creates a state of calm and relaxation. Visualization can also help us uproot negative beliefs in our subconscious by creating new neural pathways with our new, more positive beliefs, thoughts, and behavior patterns.

I recall in the early days of practicing S.T.E.P.S., I was laying in bed one night and couldn't sleep because the thought, "I am being punished by God," was flooding my mind. It became very overwhelming and I felt anxious, so I took some breaths to calm myself down. My thoughts were causing the anxiety, but before I could analyze which specific thought was causing it, I had to center myself. After taking a few deep breaths, I began to picture myself in a fetal position inside the womb of the universe. This image is my "safe place" because it reminds me that I am connected to the Creator and everything in the universe, which grounds and centers me. On my inhale, I repeated the words, "I breathe in peace and serenity," and on my exhale, I repeated, "I release all distressing thoughts." The anxiety went away and I felt a sense of calm after doing this technique.

The technique I just described is breath focus, which combines both deep breathing and visualization by the repetition of a word or phrase. Now, I want you to practice breath focus for *Stop*.

First, go to a quiet place and remove as many external distractions as possible. Before you begin, choose an image (your visualized safe space) and a word or phrase you will say as you inhale and exhale that makes you feel peaceful and safe.

When you're ready, close your eyes and begin to focus on your breathing. Just observe your inhale and exhale for a few minutes.

Next, transition to taking slow, deep breaths in and out. As you inhale, breathe in from your abdomen and then slowly release. Practice deep breathing until you get used to the shift from your normal breathing. When you are comfortable with the deep breathing, begin to picture yourself in your "safe space." If you can't think of an image, then picture yourself standing on the shore of an empty beach with gentle waves crashing. As you inhale and exhale, say the words or phrases that you chose. For example, I chose "I breathe in peace and serenity" on the inhale and "I release all distressing thoughts" on the exhale. You can continue this exercise until your mind quiets down.

Now that you have stopped the mind chatter, you are ready to move on to the next part of the S.T.E.P.S. framework, *Think*.

CHAPTER 7

Think

As we learned in Chapter 6, the beliefs in our subconscious mind influence our conscious thoughts, which affect how we feel. In turn, how we feel alters our behaviors, decisions, and actions. This is the basis of my philosophy: Transform your beliefs, transform your life. When we uproot the harmful beliefs that are shaped by toxic religious experiences and replace them with beliefs that better serve us, we produce outcomes that transform our lives for the better.

Think calls us to identify what specific thoughts and beliefs are causing us distress and creating negativity. Our emotions are a great indicator of whether our thoughts are helpful or harmful. If we think positive thoughts, then we typically feel "good," but if we think negative thoughts, it's likely to produce a "bad" mood. This does not mean we must maintain positive thoughts all the time—that would be impossible. Our goal is to take control of negative self-talk and break patterns that have become instinctive and habitual. Or else we become stuck in a perpetual cycle of negative thoughts, which leads to issues such as anxiety, depression, and low self-esteem.

At this step, we ask, "What is the thought I am having?" and "What is the underlying belief that is influencing this thought?" This is where we see just how much the toxic religious doctrine, fear, and spiritual abuse has impacted our lives. Through my healing journey, I began to think consciously about the negative thoughts and beliefs I had about myself, God, and my circumstances. I was able to see how much my negative self-talk was influenced by my experience with my mom, Billy, and the doctrine that was taught at my former church.

Religion and spirituality can provide a sense of morality, peace, solace, support, and purpose. But when the doctrine and behaviors of the community are unhealthy, we form distorted beliefs and thoughts. One example is religious fundamentalism, the strict adherence to a doctrine based on the literal interpretation of a religious text. Religious fundamentalists contend that the text is infallible and inerrant and reject ideas that contradict it. This is dangerous because it causes us to develop an elitist "us versus them" mentality and a tendency to demonize anyone or anything that conflicts with that belief. Another example is legalism—a religious doctrine that requires rigid, literal conformity to religious rules or laws. This can lead to self-righteousness and create a judgmental environment where those who do not conform are condemned.

We can be negatively influenced when we are subjected to an abuse of power in a religious community. When we accept unhealthy doctrines such as fundamentalism, legalism, or experience spiritual abuse, it becomes ingrained in our minds.

As I shared earlier in the book, I was once part of a church that was both fundamentalist and legalistic. The pastor and his wife were very controlling. The pastor often talked about living holy and abstaining from sins such as drinking, smoking, and premarital sex, urging us to distance ourselves from people who engaged in such activities. He often compared our congregation to others in the city, claiming that people in other churches were not practicing true holiness. Part of the doctrine at the church was that God had a specific plan for every person and failing to follow it meant forfeiting their blessings. His wife once told me that I should wait to get confirmation from the pastor before deciding anything. She would say, "If it's really God's will for you to do something, then He will tell your pastor."

There were even restrictions on how we dressed. For instance, women who sang on the praise team could not wear pants. One woman's daughter was told that she could no longer sing in the youth choir because she dyed her hair pink. At one point, the pastor appointed me as the leader of the media ministry. I was working as a high school teacher at the time and one day, a student asked me to come to the football game to watch him play and I agreed. When I went to church later that evening, I informed the pastor that I would not be attending a service we were having later in the week because I was going to the game. The pastor gave me a stern look and said, "I can't authorize you to miss church to go to a football game." I respectfully replied, "I was not asking permission, just informing you that I won't be there." The pastor looked at me with disgust.

I attended the game, and the following Sunday, the pastor called me into his office and said, "I like things to be done the right way, so I'm demoting you." The pastor believed that loving God meant spending the majority of your time at church, so we had church services several nights a week. In fact, the pastor or his wife would call you if you missed any service to find out why.

By the time I separated from that church, I was in a state of confusion, fear, and depression. The doctrine I had been exposed to caused me to fear that God was angry with me and had sentenced me to punishment. It also did not help that they kept trying to convince me to come back to the church by saying, "God said your place is here with us and the safest place to be is in God's will." Believing that God was punishing me caused low self-esteem and anxiety. Because I felt bad about myself and had this deep fear, I passed up opportunities thinking that I did not deserve them.

Even though I left the church, the toxic doctrine and environment had affected not only how I felt about myself, but also my decisions, behavior, and actions. So, I had to *think* about where the negative self-talk was coming from in order to change it. I identified the thought, "I am being punished by God" as part of the source of my distress.

As survivors, we have to examine how our beliefs and thoughts are influenced by our traumatic religious/spiritual experiences. This allows us to bring subconscious negative thoughts to the surface and interrupt unhealthy patterns of thoughts and behaviors. This new thinking gives us the ability to challenge them. Another benefit is that it helps us regulate our emotions because we have gained control.

Once you have *stopped* and found your center, visualize yourself grabbing hold of one of the negative thoughts you're having. Hold that thought in your hand and keep a firm grasp on it.

Now you're ready to *Evaluate!*

CHAPTER 8

Evaluate

valuate is the step where you separate the beliefs you want to hold on to from those that you want to let go of. During *think*, you grabbed hold of the thought and traced it back to its origin. Now, look at what you're holding in your hand and ask yourself, "Does this thought serve my highest good?" If the answer is no, then it would benefit you greatly to let it go.

Stephen R. Covey, author of *7 Habits of Highly Effective People*, said, "I am not a product of my circumstances. I am a product of my decisions." You determine what you need to let go of by looking at the results it has produced in your life. Are you confident or insecure? Are you depressed or happy?

We learned how repetitive thoughts make neural pathways in the brain stronger and automatic. Old habits can be hard to change, but the point is that they *can* be changed. Vance and Wright (2009) explain that initially, scientists believed that the brain was static and couldn't heal from damage or disease, but as studies of the brain progressed, it was realized that it is moldable. The writers explain, "Fortunately, scientists are becoming more aware of how malleable and plastic the brain can be. In fact, the brain has the opportunity to grow and shrink due to a process called neuroplasticity. Neuroplasticity refers to the brain's ability to change in response to environmental stimuli."[4] They make a distinction between positive neuroplasticity and negative neuroplasticity. Positive neuroplasticity occurs when the brain is stimulated by positive input and creates neural pathways that increase cognition, cognitive functioning, and produces healthy changes that create harmony between the mind

---

4. David Vance & Mary Wright, "Positive and Negative Neuroplasticity Implications for Age-related Cognitive Declines," *Journal of Gerontological Nursing* 35(6) (2009): p. 11–17, https://doi.org/10.3928/00989134-20090428-02

and body.[5] Negative neuroplasticity, on the other hand, occurs when the brain is exposed to negative stimuli, creating pathways that are harmful to the brain's functioning. Habitual patterns of negative thinking produce negative neuroplasticity. This is why it is so important to evaluate our thoughts, beliefs, and emotions so that we can take an honest look at what we need to change.

The traumas we experienced have caused dysfunction in the autonomic nervous system and emotional dysregulation, manifesting as issues such as PTSD and panic attacks. But if we reframe our thinking, the neural pathways created by our negative old thought patterns will become weak and as we practice our new thoughts and beliefs, these neural pathways will be strengthened, essentially rewiring our brains. As a result, balance will be restored to our autonomic nervous system, bringing emotional stability and improving our mental health overall.

Religious trauma can cause us to have biased thoughts that are exaggerated and irrational, known

---

5. See Footnote 4

as cognitive distortions. There are various types of cognitive distortions including the following:

- **All-or-Nothing Thinking: Viewing situations as black-and-white.**

  Example: I committed a sin by lusting after a woman at the grocery store, so that makes me a bad Christian.

- **Overgeneralization: Making broad false assumptions without evidence to support them.**

  Example: People who don't practice my religion are lost souls who don't know the true God.

- **Discounting the Positives: Dismissing positive experiences.**

  Example: It doesn't matter how much good I do, I will never be worthy of God's love.

- **Magnification (Catastrophizing) or Minimization: Blowing negative experiences out of proportion or downplaying positive events.**

  Example: A person who questions a passage from the Bible thinks, "Oh no, I am questioning my faith! I'm sinning against

God. He will never forgive me. I'm going to hell for this."

- **Must Statements: Making "must," "ought," and "should" statements that can lead to feelings of inadequacy when we don't follow through.**

   Example: Thinking, "I must follow all religious laws at all times to be holy" and feeling guilty when you don't.

Once I caught hold of my thought, "I am being punished by God," I evaluated it and saw very clearly how it affected my behavior. First, I asked myself, "Is this thought based on facts or assumptions?" I admitted to myself that what I was believing was an assumption with no evidence to support it. It was a case of all-or-nothing thinking because I was only thinking about the mistakes I made and automatically drew the conclusion that God must be mad about them. I realized that the thought was coming from the ideas that were taught at my former church.

Next, I asked, "How does holding this thought benefit or harm me?" I recognized that the thought was harming me because it caused me to develop low self-esteem, depression, anxiety, and suicidal ideations. I felt helpless and hopeless and was afraid of taking chances in life because I didn't believe I was worthy of happiness. Next, I asked myself, "Does this thought serve my highest good?" The answer was no, so I knew this belief was something that I needed to release and reframe because the distress I was experiencing was directly related to what I was believing and telling myself.

The first step in your reframing is to stop and the next step is to think about what specific thought is causing your distress and grab hold of it. When you have a firm grasp of that thought, ask yourself the following questions:

1. Is this thought based on facts or assumptions?

2. What evidence supports or contradicts this thought?

3. How does holding this thought benefit or harm me?

4. What would I tell a friend who has this thought?

5. Does this thought serve my highest good?

This step calls for deep self-reflection on the negative thoughts and behavioral patterns that keep us stuck. *Evaluation* is an empowering process because we find the courage to take charge of our lives by facing painful experiences from our pasts to bring healing and resolution. We build strength, resilience, gain wisdom, and rediscover ourselves through this process.

Although *evaluation* is an important step, I want to restate that some things such as sexual abuse may be too painful to confront on your own. In such cases, please evaluate that thought with a therapist.

You have grabbed hold of the thought and evaluated it, now you can *Pivot*.

CHAPTER 9

Pivot

This is when the reframing begins. In *Pivot*, you take the negative thought that you evaluated and turn away from it by changing it into something that serves you in a more positive or useful way. In Chapter 8, we learned that cognitive distortions are the false beliefs we carry with us. We explored how our perceptions of reality have been distorted by the thoughts and beliefs that we have formed based on our negative religious or spiritual experiences. If we don't *pivot*, we will be stuck in that negative loop, which, if it continues, may lead to a more severe mental challenge like psychosis. When we *pivot*, however, we replace those negative thoughts and beliefs with a perspective that is more helpful.

We also learned about neuroplasticity—the brain's ability to change by the neural pathways that are formed by our thoughts, beliefs, and things that we learn. Since our brains have been wired by our negative religious experiences, we effectively rewire our brains by forming new neural pathways. This is done by replacing the negative thoughts and beliefs with positive thoughts and beliefs through *pivoting*. The more we practice this, the more it balances our autonomic nervous system and brings us into a state of calm so we can think clearly and make rational decisions.

One research study showed how positive visual reframing helped participants cope with disturbing negative experiences and regulate their emotional responses. "When attempts to understand and explain the meaning of a negative experience are successful, we generally find closure and move on. Otherwise, the experience remains 'open' and is easily triggered by reminiscent experiences and emotional and visual cues," explained the researchers.[6] Participants were asked to recall an experience that held strong negative emotions for them. Through the reframing technique, they were able to resolve their distress and find balance. Eiroa-Orosa and Ruppert wrote, "Findings suggest [positive visual reframing] provides an efficient and functional emotional regulation strategy when negative emotions are triggered. It is further suggested that in defusing a perceptual threat, [positive visual reframing] might free cognitive space to enable fresh insight to arise and potentially unseat rigidly held negative perceptions."[7] Their research on positive visual reframing shows us that reframing is a powerful tool that not only benefits brain functioning and the mind, but is a life-changing process in general.

Pivoting changes the way we see ourselves, our circumstances, others, and the world around us. We have been looking at ourselves through lenses that have been distorted by religious trauma.

---

6. Ruppert, J. C., & Eiroa-Orosa, F. J. (2018). Positive visual reframing: A randomised controlled trial using drawn visual imagery to defuse the intensity of negative experiences and regulate emotions in healthy adults. *Anales de Psicología*, 34(2), 368–376. https://www.researchgate.net/publication/324598245_Positive_visual_reframing_A_randomised_controlled_trial_using_drawn_visual_imagery_to_defuse_the_intensity_of_negative_experiences_and_regulate_emotions_in_healthy_adults

7. See Footnote 6.

As we reframe our thinking, we will start to see ourselves in a more positive light and feel better about ourselves. It will also change the way we view situations and our position in life from pessimism to optimism. We begin to see hope where we felt hopeless and begin to see light where, before, we only saw darkness. As we establish autonomy, we are able to open ourselves to healthy relationships that are based on mutual respect and honesty. We can let our guard down and begin to feel safe and secure in the world.

When I analyzed the thought, "I am being punished by God" and evaluated how it was affecting my self-esteem, feelings, behavior, decisions, and actions, I knew it was time to *pivot*. I could see how this belief was causing me to be stuck and unable to move forward due to fear and depression. Being clear on my thought of "I am being punished by God" has allowed me to see that I had a distorted perception. In my pivoting, I realized I was not disfavored by God. I finally understood that even though I experienced some unfavorable situations, they did not define who I was. I reframed my thought from "I am being punished by God" to "I am a survivor."

Making that pivot was a life-changing moment—I felt lighter, like a weight had been lifted. I realized that my life was not "ruined." Rather, I had unlimited opportunities before me, and I was free to make choices without fear of God's wrath. I began to recognize that I deserved good things and started to expect positive outcomes.

You grabbed ahold of your negative thought and evaluated it to see how it has impacted you. You recognized that it does not serve your highest good, so now, let's *pivot*. Close your eyes and imagine you are holding the thought in your hand again. Imagine a trash can sitting beside you, and when you're ready, throw the thought away. You recognize that the thought was an assumption that was not based on facts. Now, replay a situation in your mind in which your negative thought showed up, and this time, look for evidence that contradicts that thought. Think of a way to interpret the situation that is more positive—reframe your thought. Next, take a few deep breaths and meditate on the new thought for a moment—let it sink into your mind.

This is not a one and done process because your negative thoughts and beliefs have been running non-stop. So, you will find those thoughts and beliefs coming up again and again. When they do, use the reframed thought that you came up with to challenge them. Another technique is to say the reframed thought to yourself throughout the day as a reminder. Journaling can also be a helpful tool for reflection during the reframing process. As you continue to practice reframing, the new thought will create new neural pathways which will grow stronger through repetition while the old neural pathways grow weaker as the negative thoughts and beliefs change.

Pivoting empowers you because it helps you regain control of your mind after experiencing religious trauma. As we learned in Chapter 6, we have thousands of thoughts per day. However, we don't have to be prisoners to our thoughts. Instead, we have the power to choose the ones on which to focus. Like watering a garden, the ones that we focus on will grow. So, *pivoting* helps us uproot the negative thoughts and beliefs that become embedded in the subconscious mind. When we reframe, we plant new positive thoughts into the garden of our minds.

Now that we have *pivoted*, we are able to move on to the next step where we begin to *see* things more clearly.

CHAPTER 10

See

Working through the S.T.E.P.S. is a cathartic process that helps us free ourselves from unhealthy habitual thoughts and belief patterns caused by religious trauma. It allows us to establish autonomy and values that align with our true selves and live lives of purpose and fulfillment. A process such as this requires introspection, which brings us to our final step, *see*.

See is where we look at how we feel after we've *pivoted* and reframed our thoughts. Trauma affects our whole being—mind, body, and soul, and it is important to note how the changes we make as we progress benefit our well-being along our healing journey. Pay attention to the difference between how you felt previously and how you feel after you *pivot*. As we have been learning in this book, how we think affects how we feel, so thinking differently should lead to feeling differently. Knowing the difference between how we were before reframing and how we are now allows us to recognize the power we have to overcome our trauma. This allows us to take back our power and never succumb to those negative thoughts again.

It is important to pay attention to how we feel during *see* because there are deep, strong emotions tied to memories of painful experiences. It is only when we work through those painful experiences that we are able to heal from them and resolve those negative emotions. When we are healed, those memories do not evoke the same intense emotional impact as they once did so we are able to *see* the difference. The research study we discussed in Chapter 9 provides an example of how introspection is an essential part of the healing process. Eiroa-Orosa and Ruppert's study is significant because they understood that negative memories "contain high levels of emotional detail, emotional significance, and information, which when combined greatly increases the likelihood the memory will be maintained," and so hypothesized that reframing would help the participants resolve their negative feelings and reduce their level of intensity and impact on their well-being.[8] The participants were tested on the intensity of their negative memory prior to performing the reframing exercise and then retested after completing it. The testing and retesting were a crucial aspect of the study because it allowed the researchers and participants to *see* the before and after results. The results indicated that the level of intensity of their negative feelings dropped after reframing just as Ruppert and Eiroa-Orosa hypothesized.[9] Their findings show us that a reframing process like S.T.E.P.S. works and the results will be undeniable—we will *see* the evidence because we will feel better.

I have broken the S.T.E.P.S. down into chapters, but it is a process that flows seamlessly together when put into action. This framework shows

---

8. Francisco Eiroa-Orosa and Julia Ruppert, "Positive visual reframing: A randomised controlled trial using drawn visual imagery to defuse the intensity of negative experiences and regulate emotions in healthy adults," *Anales de Psicología* 34(2) (2018): p. 368–376, https://doi.org/10.6018/analesps.34.2.286191

9. See Footnote 8

you how to deconstruct the negative religious programming that is robbing you of your peace and keeping you from reaching your potential. If you are experiencing anxiety, depression, or some other form of distress due to religious trauma and you follow the format—stop, think, evaluate, pivot, you will start to *see* your mental state improve.

Seeing my transformation was a massive relief and gave me a sense of pride. My self-esteem skyrocketed and even my everyday behavior was more positive. I no longer felt anxiety when applying for jobs because I had developed confidence in myself and my skills, so I knew I was well-qualified. The fear and confusion about knowing God's plan for me went away and I was able to think clearly and make sound decisions. When I stopped believing that God was punishing me, I recognized that the only thing holding me back was myself. The feelings of hopelessness and helplessness left because I realized that my perception creates my reality and I refused to be controlled by self-doubt and self-loathing any longer. I found the will and determination to live and the courage to dream again and set goals. I recognized that I was passionate about mental health and inner healing so I began to pursue a career in the mental health field.

I forgave myself for my past mistakes and released the resentment and anger I had toward those who hurt me. This made room in my heart to form reciprocal relationships based on warmth, acceptance, and love with people whose intentions were for my highest good. Once I understood that my thoughts influenced my behavior and how I felt, I became more conscious of the thoughts I allowed into my mind. This framework is the tool I have used over and over again, and even now, and I am blessed enough to share it with other people.

*****

As I am writing this, I am overjoyed as I reflect on how far I have come in my healing journey. *Seeing* is not just about noticing the difference in the way we feel, it is also about acknowledging how we've grown and celebrating what we've overcome. As you work the S.T.E.P.S. to your healing, do not forget to celebrate, even the small wins. This is how we encourage ourselves to keep going because we see how we are being transformed.

Take a small pause by closing your eyes and breathing deeply. Observe how you previously felt and compare it to how you feel now. It may take a bit of time to train your brain to shift your thoughts to a more positive state. It's okay if you do not feel a drastic change at first. Each time the negative thought creeps back in, work the S.T.E.P.S. again as much and as long as you need to, and once the shift does happen, you will see the difference. You will make progress as you continue the process. If you keep working the S.T.E.P.S., you will see the world differently. That's what Transformative Spiritual Coaching is about—empowering people with tools to recover from religious trauma and seeing their lives transform for the better. That is my mission.

If this book has impacted you, then I invite you to join my support group, connect with me on social media, or email me by scanning the QR code at the end of this book.

CHAPTER 11

Maintaining Your Peace

Setting Boundaries

Now that you have worked through the S.T.E.P.S., you should have a better understanding of some of the things that trigger distress. Knowing what makes you uncomfortable helps you to establish the parameters of your boundaries. You can draw the line that you don't want anyone to cross, and you will be able to recognize when someone violates that boundary.

Be firm about your boundaries because you are essentially doing what is necessary to maintain your peace. When you have not set boundaries in the past, it may be difficult for some to accept the change. They may get angry or act as if you have committed a great transgression. Do not let anyone guilt you into thinking that taking care of yourself is wrong. Stick to your boundaries and be consistent.

When someone attempts to hold a discussion with you about something that causes you agony, it is okay to let the person know that you do not want to talk about it without giving a lengthy explanation as to why. For example, you might say, "I understand that your beliefs are important to you, but I do not want to discuss it." Another example is to say, "I hear what you are saying, but I would rather not discuss it." You also have the right to walk away if the person dismisses what you say and tries to force the conversation. Certain religious holidays, rituals, or services may give you discomfort. If so, you are entitled to say, "No, I do not want to participate," rather than doing something that makes you uneasy to please others or avoid ridicule.

Finally, prioritize your well-being and spiritual journey. It's okay to distance yourself from those who are harmful to your progress.

Finding Your New Spiritual Path

The adverse religious or spiritual experience from your past may cause you to be leery about becoming affiliated with another religious or spiritual group, and your reservations are valid. You can explore other spiritual philosophies and religions without committing to anything, and there are various ways to do so. You can start by reading books, watching videos, and listening to podcasts on subjects that interest you. Another way is to interact with online communities and forums to gain information. You can also attend a class or workshop in person or virtually to learn more.

While exploring different spiritual or religious systems, you can adopt the ideals that resonate with you without fully adopting the entire belief system. It's about finding practices and rituals that make you feel connected to the Universe and others.

Remember, be weary of people who attempt to force you to think the same way they do or adopt the practices that they have for the sake of assimilating.

Rebuilding Your Community

We are not meant to live in this world by ourselves, but you may be finding it hard to trust again. Being supported by loving people who make you feel safe can help facilitate your healing. There are empathic support groups, like mine, that provide a welcoming environment. You can also establish connections with people who have similar lifestyle choices like bonding at a yoga studio or book club. Connect with people who respect your boundaries and help you feel secure and supported.

Getting to Know the Real You

First and foremost, you are not a victim, you are victorious! You may feel like you lost yourself through that negative religious or spiritual experience, and that can be scary and confusing. I am here to tell you that you are going to be okay. When you start to deconstruct those negative thoughts and beliefs, you are peeling off the layers to get to the "real" you. As you get rid of the toxic ideology, you can begin to define what you truly value and stand for. When you stop basing your decisions and actions on the opinions of an unhealthy religious or spiritual leader and community, you can begin to ask yourself, "What do I truly want?" and listen to your heart. Pay attention to what motivates you and ignites you passionately. What are you naturally drawn to? What piques your curiosity? And ask yourself, "Why?"

Part of my philosophy is: Life is a school and experience is our teacher. I do not believe in coincidences—I believe that everything that happens is meant to happen. I see each experience, whether we view it as good or bad, as an opportunity to learn and grow. Even when we experience adversity, we go through it and come out on the other side wiser and stronger. If I had not gone through religious trauma, I would not be a religious trauma expert and coach, nor would I be writing this book. This is how I made meaning out of the things that I have suffered in the past. As you work through your religious trauma, pay attention to the things that you discover about yourself. What new revelations are you getting as you heal and recover? What positive changes are you making as you work through the S.T.E.P.S.? Look for the silver lining in what you went through.

Journaling is an effective way to express and sort out your thoughts and feelings. Meditation can also help you gain clarity and get more in tune with your intuition. Reading and hearing other people's stories of how they overcame adversity can be encouraging and help us make meaning of and reflect on our own experiences. Lastly, when we are ready, sharing our stories in a supportive environment can be therapeutic and liberating, helping us see how far we've come. Celebrate your progress and what you have overcome.

Final Thoughts

As we reach the end of this book, I want to congratulate you for the courage and resilience you've shown every step of the way. Healing from religious trauma requires confronting painful memories and challenging deeply ingrained beliefs. But it is a process which is necessary to bring about true transformation in our lives.

The S.T.E.P.S. to Freedom Framework is designed to guide you to healing and transformation with empathy and compassion. I hope that it has been useful in helping you to reclaim your identity, heal your wounds, and redefine your spirituality.

Thank you for allowing me to be a part of your growth and recovery process. I want you to know that you are brave, you are strong, and you are worthy of a life filled with happiness. You have already taken significant steps toward healing by reading this book and engaging with the S.T.E.P.S. Embrace your journey with confidence, knowing that you have the power to transform your beliefs and, ultimately, your life. You've got this!

Peace, love, and light!

About The Author

Ivory's life transformation began in 2010 after suffering a nervous breakdown. It brought her to the realization that she had unresolved trauma that she needed to heal. The road to healing led Ivory to face the painful experiences of abuse from her childhood and how the pattern had continued in her life. The unresolved trauma manifested as depression, anxiety, low self-esteem, shame, guilt, suicidal ideations, and spiritual crisis. Left unresolved, the symptoms became so severe that she had to be hospitalized. This is when things began to turn around for Ivory. Prior to being hospitalized, she knew that she didn't feel good about herself, but Ivory did not know how to change that. Through therapy, she learned coping skills and was equipped with tools to help her heal. Ivory also learned that negative self-talk was the root of what was causing her to feel bad about herself and began to reframe her thoughts and beliefs. As she began to transform her beliefs about herself, Ivory's whole life changed. Overcoming these mental and emotional challenges inspired her to help others who are experiencing such challenges and develop her own powerful framework. Ivory now teaches others how to overcome mental and emotional pain that prevents them from living a fulfilled life through her S.T.E.P.S. to Freedom Method. As a spiritual coach, she believes that true healing encompasses the total self—mind, body, and spirit, and her role is to help you find what makes you feel aligned and rooted in your identity so that you find purpose and fulfillment in life.

Ivory received training as a spiritual coach through the Life Purpose Institute, Kemetic Centered Living, Integrative Mental Health University, and Transformation Academy, and she continues to learn, study, and develop her skills. Prior to becoming a spiritual coach, Ivory worked in several areas of the mental health field including peer support, substance abuse, applied behavior analysis, and employment support. She earned her bachelor's degree in Broadcast Journalism from Langston University in 2002 and has taken graduate courses in spiritual counseling and applied behavior analysis.

Today, Ivory is dedicated to helping others conquer their mental and emotional turmoil through her S.T.E.P.S. to Freedom Method. As a spiritual coach, she believes that true healing integrates the mind, body, and spirit. Her mission is to help you uncover your true identity, align with your deepest values, and live a life filled with purpose and fulfillment.

www.ingramcontent.com/pod-product-compliance
Lightning Source LLC
Chambersburg PA
CBHW062227150726 ·
47991CB00006B/2471